ANGELA MOWERY

Herbs for Emotional Support

A Holistic Approach for Sufferers of Stress, Anxiety and Depression

Contents

1

Introduction

Are you feeling down, stressed, depressed, or sleepless? If so, certain plants can probably help alleviate these feelings. Aromas from plants are some of the most amazing pick-me-ups that cost very little, if anything. Plants have been used by many herbalists for thousands of years to heal and stay healthy. In fact, there are many books throughout history where herbal medicine is discussed. Herbal remedies can not only help with symptoms of an ailment, but also prevent any future diseases or help with other illnesses as a bonus.

There are a couple of benefits to using herbal medicine. First, it's affordable. Rather than a medication that costs a hundred dollars or more, herbs are rather cheap. They are even cheaper if you grow them yourself in your backyard or in a pot on the windowsill. Another benefit is that there are not as many side effects from taking a natural remedy. Have you ever seen a commercial about a drug and at the end, there are a whole list of side effects? It makes someone question why to take that specific drug. Herbs don't really have that issue. Now with that being said, they are not regulated as medicine by the FDA in the United States. Other countries may have different regulations on herbs that i am not familiar with. So do your research before using. Taking natural remedies while also taking conventional medications could cause some very serious side effects. I am not a doctor and do not claim that herbs are the way to go for all people. Please consult a licensed doctor before embarking on a natural health journey to make sure that no complications will arise. If your symptoms are severe, say to the point that you have trouble functioning, please also consult a doctor immediately rather than going the herbal route. Unfortunately, herbs can only do so much to help manage a symptom.

This is a small guide that I came up with on five plants that can help with emotional support and well-being. Some of these are well known and a couple of them might be new to you. They are all acknowledged in the herbal community as being calming in nature. Please use this as a guide as everybody is different and what works for one, may not work for another. In other words, do your research and determine if it may be useful to you and fits into your lifestyle. Say, for instance, you feel that tea would be beneficial to you. If you do not have the time to brew the tea though, then maybe that won't be the best form for you to use. If you have pets, then diffusing an essential oil in the air is not recommended as some oils cause complications with pets. The same as with people, each animal is different and may have unforeseen reactions. Do not use herbs on a child, especially babies and toddlers, without doing some research. Some oils should not be used at all and others should be used in smaller doses. Again, if unsure, please check with a pediatrician to see if a particular herb is able to be used on your child. Do not go to the internet and search as there are many different variables and/or misinformation that will be found out there.

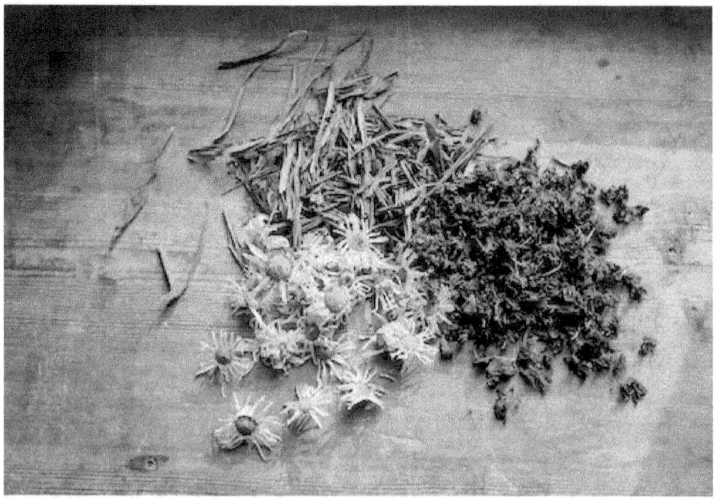

Dried herbs

2

Research

When buying herbs, especially an essential oil, know what to look for on the label. Labels should be clear and concise. They should have the manufacturer information shown as well as a contact number. Some essential oils may be a blend of different oils rather than just the one oil that you are thinking it is. This makes them a little less expensive to produce. The label should indicate the different ingredients and the Latin name as well as the country of origin. Labels can also show that it is a supplement, but cannot make any health claims about treating a disease or healing a condition. Supplements are not standardized, meaning that there is not any testing across the board for uniformity. One brand could be 100% what it says, while another could only be 85% and the other 15% is filler. For this reason, I try to avoid supplements unless I have vetted the brand completely and trust them.

Some herbs can cause allergic reactions in certain individuals. Specifically, those with seasonal allergies such as hay fever, should not use anything in the aster or daisy family of plants, including chamomile. This will just aggravate your allergies even more and discourage the use of natural plants in the future. Also, some plants can cause adverse effects on your health. As an example, St. John's Wort interacts with multiple different medications, so if you are considering taking it, get with your doctor first and make sure that it is fine to use. This is on repeat throughout this book because it is an important piece of information. If you have medical issues, and plan on taking herbal medicine, your conventional doctor needs to know. This is where research and communication with your doctor comes into play to help guide you.

3

Ways to Use

There are multiple ways to use herbs in daily preparations or as needed. One of the most common is taken as a tea. Walk down the tea aisle of any grocery store and you will see many varieties of herbal teas. This is one of my preferred ways of using herbs. It's a running joke around my house that I have more types of tea than anything else in my kitchen. There are also tinctures, which are fresh herbs steeped usually in an alcohol or vegetable glycerin base for a couple of months and then strained. These are extremely potent and not because of the alcohol. The alcohol evaporates enough that it becomes a non-issue. The potency comes from the oils that are derived directly from the fresh leaves. Supplements are usually pills and can be found in or around the vitamin section of a store. These are usually dried and powdered versions of an herb. As mentioned previously though, there is no guarantee that they are exactly what they say in the description. There are infused products available that include herbal components in them. Shampoos and lotions come to mind specifically but there are also salves and balms. Most of these are bath and body related.

Essential oils are a huge part of the herbal community. In a nutshell, the plant will go through a distillation process that extracts the pure oil from the plant. One bottle of essential oil is made from several pounds of this plant. The extract, or scent, is then bottled up and marketed as essential oil. This is a potent form as it is pure and should be used with caution. The oil is used in aromatherapy where it is diffused into the air, inhaled or used on the skin. An essential oil should not be placed directly on the skin. Placing directly on the skin has the potential to cause a reaction. Dilute it in what is called a carrier oil, such as olive, coconut or almond oils, and use as a massage oil. Some will take an essential oil internally for some reason or another. Personally, I do not do this. Since there are no regulations, that kind of makes me nervous about what I am putting in my body. Plus some oils are not to be ingested at all. If you choose to go this route, then make sure that they are food grade, it should say somewhere on the bottle. As a note, fragrance oils are not essential oils. That is a whole different process and are usually made with synthetic chemicals besides plant oils.

4

Dosages

When it comes to dosing on herbal products, caution should be used. Guidelines for dosing herbal concoctions vary greatly. While herbal teas can be drank everyday, they should not be consumed more than three times a day. This will help avoid any side effects. Tinctures should start off at about 15-20 drops, either added to a small cup of water or dropped directly into the mouth. If the tincture is being taken by a child or an elderly adult, then this should be reduced considerably depending on age. Dosing of tinctures is not a "one size fits all". Dosage is specific to each person, depending on size of person, why it is being taken plus if any reactions are involved in larger doses with said person. Supplements should be taken as noted on the bottle. These are all guidelines and will vary depending on the person.

Now that all of that is out of the way, let's get to the herbs!

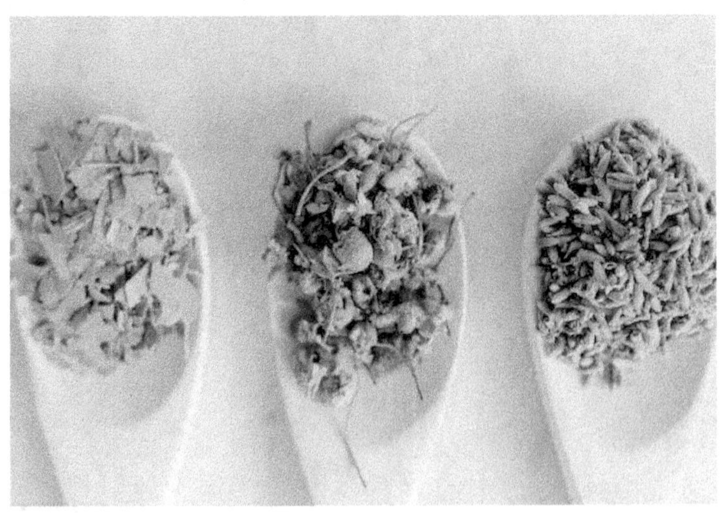

5

Lavender

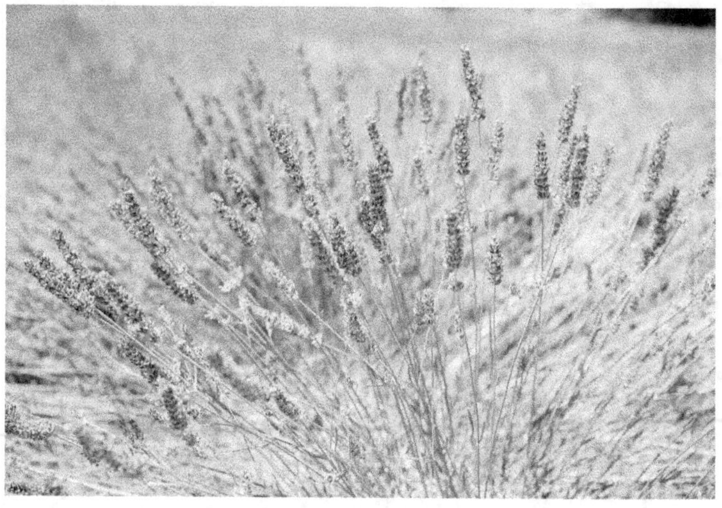

avender

L Who hasn't heard of lavender and its soothing effects?
The scent of lavender gives a sense of calm and helps
relieve tension and stress. It is one of the most common herbs

and the scent is recognizable around the world. It is used in not only perfume, but also in aromatherapy and relaxation practices. There are many varieties of lavender with the most common being English lavender (*Lavandula angustifolia*) and French lavender (*Lavandula stoechas*). The plant is stunning when grown in a large mass. I have seen pictures of lavender farms and they are beautiful. It is just a stretch of purple flowers for as far as the eye can see. I can just imagine that there is hardly any stress in that environment and the smell is divine.

Historically, lavender has been used for many things including perfume, incense, cleaning aids, and insect repellant. Medicinally, it was used as a treatment for nervousness, aches, pains, and coughs. It was also used to disinfect areas such as medical wards and doctor offices, anywhere that catered to the sick basically.

There are many scientific studies involving lavender. Most of them have studied the effects on sleep and relaxation. It has been noted that there is compelling evidence for it to be used against depression and restlessness. The aroma is known to reduce nervousness and improve mental stimulation in a maternity setting so that new mothers and babies can bond better and help with postpartum issues such as depression. Nervous systems also seem to balance themselves out with the help of lavender.

Several benefits are associated with the use of lavender. It has anti-inflammatory properties, so it is good for pain and inflammation, such as headaches. As mentioned above, there are significant advantages to using it for nervous systems. It can help reduce heart rate and normalize breathing during a panic attack. Mentally, the reduction of stress, depression and anxiety have been observed during studies. This in turn probably has an effect on the sleep pattern of an individual. Lavender is very popular as a natural sleep aid and used for insomnia.

Products containing lavender can be found in abundance. It is a very popular ingredient and well loved by many. From lotions and creams to candles, there is a product for most everybody. The scent is even used in baby products to help calm fussy infants. There is essential oil, which is commonly used for various applications. Then there are the dried products, which come in the form of tea and sachets. It can be found in cleaning products due to the antibacterial properties it possesses. So the next time you reach for that disinfectant, know that there is a reason that lavender is in that bottle for other than the scent.

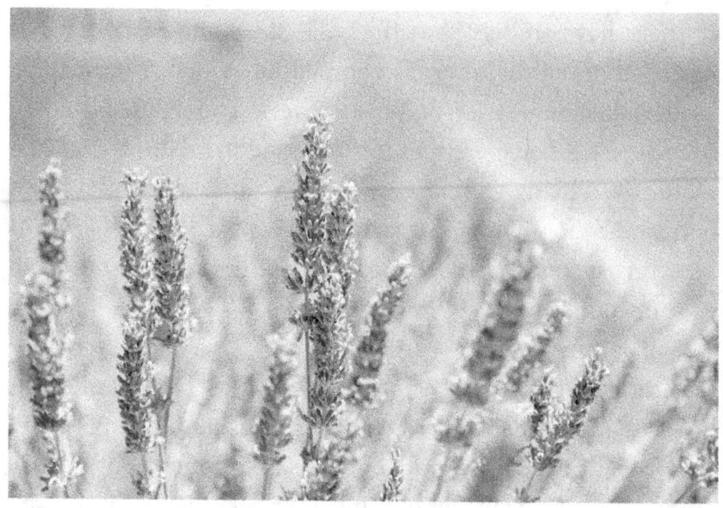

Lavender

Sleep routines involving lavender usually result in a good night's rest. Studies imply that it improves sleep quality and promotes relaxation. A spray can be made or bought using lavender that can be used on the bedding to initiate a restful night. Sachets can be filled with lavender buds and put under a pillow or sewn into a pillowcase. The pressure from sleeping on it will crush the buds and release the scent which will help with the relaxation process and insomnia.

Meditation and yoga practices use the aroma for relaxation and stress reduction. This helps set the mood for meditating and facilitate a calming effect for concentration. Usually this is done through a diffuser or as incense where the scent is dispersed throughout the area. If it is an individual and not a group setting, then the oil may be added to a necklace or directly onto the skin on pulse points using a carrier oil such as almond oil.

The oil is used in bath and body products extensively. Not only does it support emotional well-being but it is a benefit to the skin. The anti-inflammatory properties will help with skin rashes and help relieve pain in joints. Massage oils are fantastic for this reason. When used on fussy babies lavender scented baby lotions and oils help calm them down, especially if they are colicky. This helps them sleep better. There are also bath salts on the market that can be used to soak in for a relaxing atmosphere while bathing. Natural deodorants use lavender in them for the antifungal and antibacterial properties which happens to be an added benefit on top of the calming support.

Lavender is considered a safe herb to use with little to no issues in regards to interactions and allergies when used correctly. However, as with anything, there may be exceptions. If you find that you feel worse after using lavender, stop using it and talk to your doctor. Do not take it if you are pregnant or breastfeeding.

6

Mint

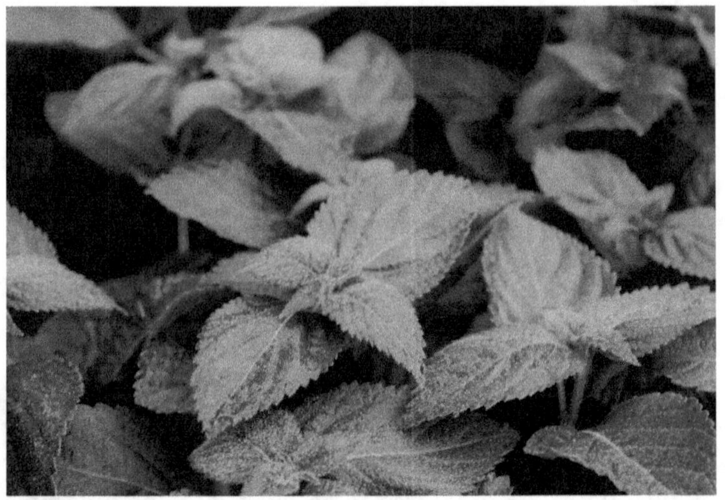

P*eppermint*

Everybody probably knows the scent of mint. Think of

candy canes, chewing gum and toothpaste. While those might freshen your breath, there are other aspects of mint that help with emotional well-being. It is a common herb although maybe not as well known as lavender when it comes to healing. However, there is history, going back as far as 1550 B.C., of mint being used by ancient Greeks, Romans and Egyptians. Since mint seems to have originated along the Mediterranean, it makes sense that those ancient cultures would have used it. While it doesn't seem to have been used for emotional purposes, it was still a valuable resource for stomach ailments, colds and even hiccups.

There are scientific studies and research that show health benefits when using mint. Of these, there is the ability to ease migraines and tension headaches. Evidence also shows that mint tea may help with sinus issues. It has not yet been determined if it is actually the properties of the mint, or just the warm steam, that does the work. In my opinion, peppermint tea tastes great so either way, it's a win. There are studies that show that the scent not only energizes and reduces fatigue but also can improve cognitive functions like memory and concentration.

When it comes to mint, there are a lot of varieties out there. The most popular are spearmint (*Mentha spicata*) and peppermint (*Mentha x piperita*).These are the scents that most people are familiar with. There are also apple, chocolate, and pineapple mints, the list goes on and on. Other plants that are related to mint that you may not think of are basil, sage, oregano, bee balm, lemon balm and thyme to name a few. The majority of mint plants like to spread all over the garden if not controlled.

I know this from experience and now grow the different plants in pots.

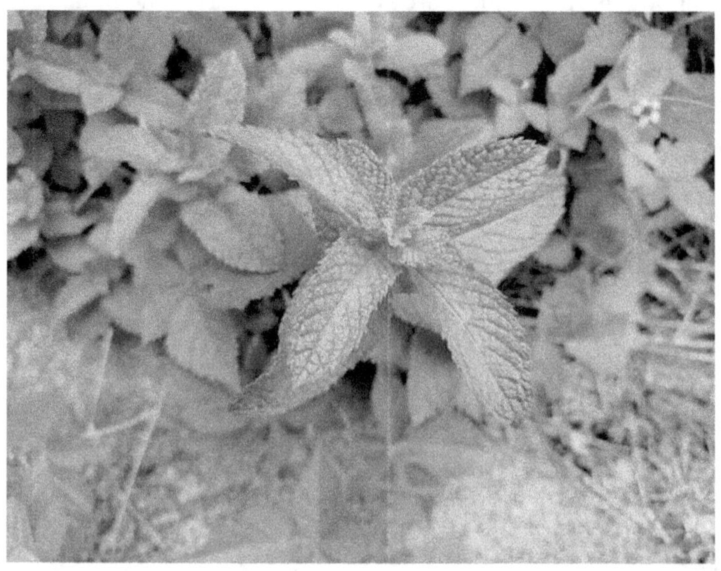

Spearmint

Mint is used in food and beverages, bath and body products and as an essential oil. It is an ingredient in mouthwash, toothpaste and hair products among other things and provides an invigorating scent to these items. Tea blends containing mint are also popular. It is one of my favorite teas and helps clear my mind when I need to focus on a task. The essential oil can be used in a diffuser so that the scent is distributed throughout an area. The aroma of mint is a revitalizing and uplifting scent. It helps clear sinuses and relieve headaches besides providing an energy boost. Personally, I use a roll-on blend consisting of peppermint and lavender oils for this specific reason. Of course, to be safe, those oils are mixed with a light oil such as almond oil so that there are no adverse effects on my skin. All I do is roll it onto my temples or the back of my neck depending on where my headache seems to be the worst.

There are not many side effects when used properly. Do not use it on pets or their bedding as it is toxic to them. As usual, if you are pregnant or nursing, please consult with your doctor before using. Also, do not use it on children or infants. There are some medical conditions that it may affect, including certain liver diseases. If you are unsure, talk to your doctor or even a pharmacist.

7

Bergamot

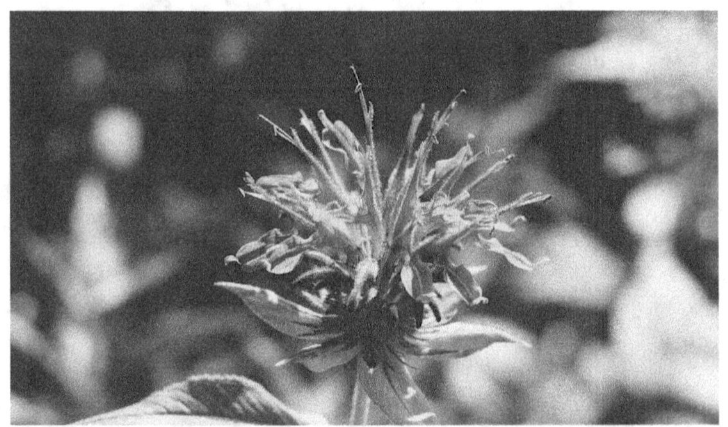

ee Balm (Wild Bergamot)

Bergamot (*Citrus bergamia*), also known as bee balm for
the wild version, is one of my favorite plants and scents

in my garden. The plant has beautiful, colorful flowers that attract bees and butterflies that give off a happy vibe. True cultured bergamot is a type of fruit that grows on trees in tropical areas and has a citrusy scent. It is a small knobby fruit that is extremely bitter tasting so don't try to incorporate it into your food. The oil is extracted from this fruit and that is the component of the plant that is used.

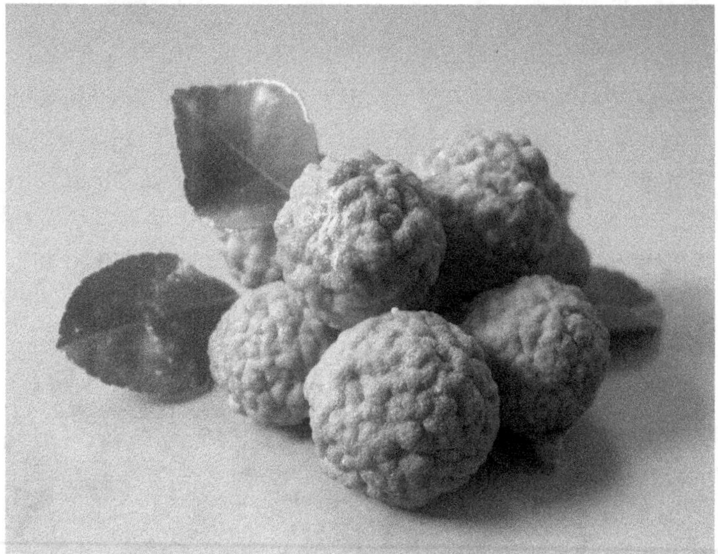

Bergamot fruit

If you drink Earl Grey tea, then you will recognize the scent of bergamot. The oil is in the tea which provides a boost to your mood. This is a good way to get a day started and, hopefully, walk away with a sense of happiness. Bergamot oil is a great rejuvenating scent when feelings of irritability or depression arise. Clinical studies have been done with aromatherapy and its effects on stress, anxiety and depression. The majority of the studies came back with positive results in reducing the conditions.

When it comes to using bergamot, other than drinking it in Earl Grey tea, it is not recommended to consume it. I have never seen anything else that contains bergamot, at least none that I can think of, that would be ingested. It is mostly used in aromatherapy and body products, such as incense, perfumes, colognes and lotions. This is one of my favorite scents for when I am feeling a bit down. I diffuse a bit of the oil into the air and inhale it for a quick burst of cheerfulness. I also have a candle infused with the scent that I will light for that sense of euphoria. When I smell it, I feel like I am standing on a beach with the sun shining down on me and waves crashing around. That is my sense of bliss and it makes me almost instantaneously happy every time.

Safety precautions that should be considered when using bergamot include avoiding exposure to sunlight. As with most citrus oils, bergamot contains a compound that makes it light sensitive. This can cause a serious skin reaction, even when diluted. There is also a chance that the oil can cause an allergic reaction when applied to the skin. This would show as a rash, blisters or even as a burning sensation. If this happens, wash the area well and quit using the product. The oil is generally considered safe for aromatherapy with pregnant women. It is still a good idea to check with your doctor though.

8

Lemon Balm

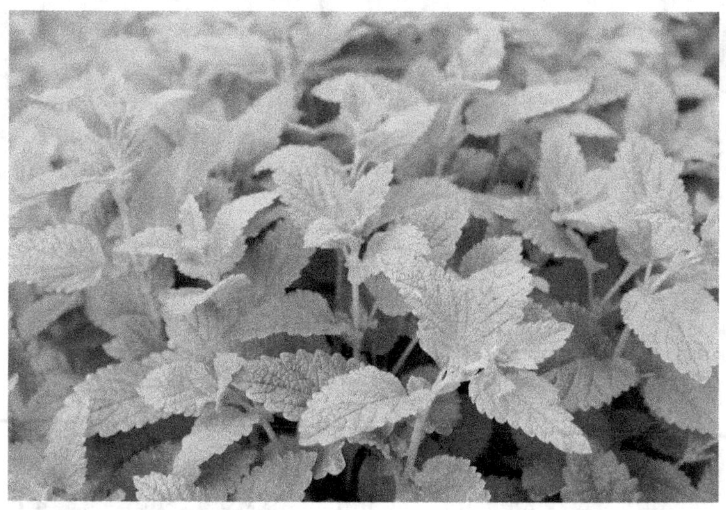

emon Balm

Lemon balm (*Melissa officinalis*) is exactly what it says. It is a balm to the senses that smells like lemony mint. This is my absolute favorite plant to grow in the garden. I love brushing up against it and releasing the scent. I love it so much that I actually don't want to pull up any volunteers that have spread out of the area where it is planted. Usually, I just dig it up and start a new garden bed elsewhere for it. Thankfully, that is only every couple of years or so, Otherwise, I would run out of room! It is a member of the mint family but doesn't seem to spread as drastically as other forms of mint.

History indicates that the plant has been used for centuries medicinally, including for mental health. Scientists indicate that there are promising studies on the plant regarding mental health, insomnia and digestive issues. The compounds in lemon balm have antioxidant, antibacterial and antimicrobial properties. This means that it is a powerhouse in medical terms and can help with various infections and viruses. For most people, this would be a safe, natural medical choice for a cold. Lemon balm has the capability of reducing stress, anxiety, depression and insomnia or other sleep issues. There is also a chance that it could help with memory and focus.

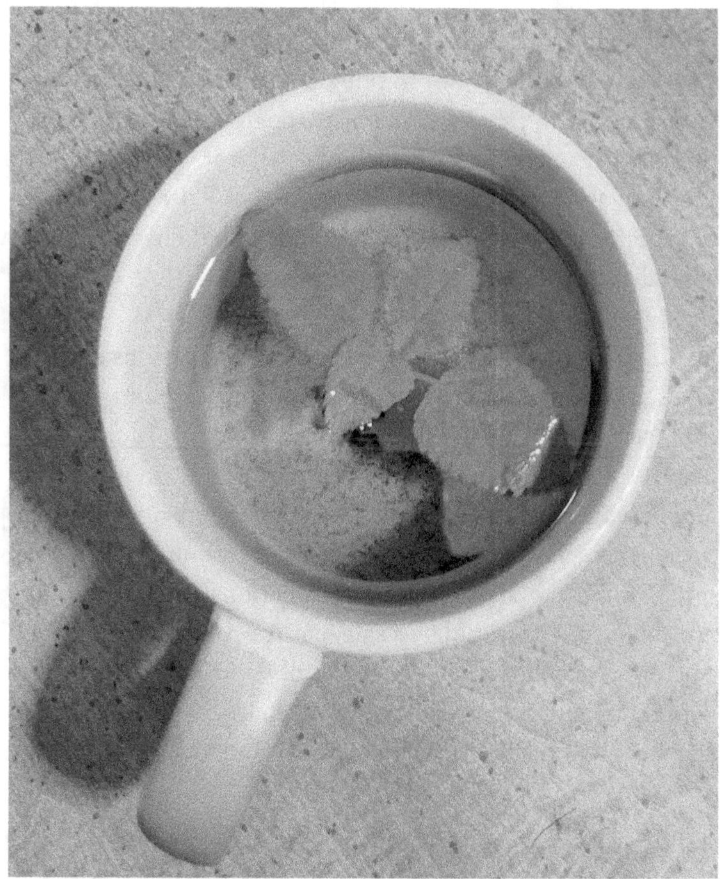

Lemon Balm tea

Tea is my choice on how I like to use lemon balm when it is needed. I have made it from both fresh leaves and dried. It smells and tastes good, plus I get calming benefits from it. Usually, I drink it later in the day closer to bedtime. It gives me a sense of relaxation and soothes any anxiety left over from the day. Drinking it before bedtime helps me fall asleep also since it has a mild sedative effect.

Other forms of lemon balm include tinctures, aromatherapy, bath and body products, and adding it to food dishes. I've never added it to food, so I can't vouch for it there. I do have a tincture where, on really bad days, I take a few drops. A little bit goes a long way when using tinctures. Aromatherapy wise, I do not have an essential oil to diffuse. However, as mentioned previously, I have fresh plants and get my aroma fixation while walking by the plants and running my hand through them. This not only gives me the scent immediately but later, when I go back inside, I still have the scent on my skin until washed off. Diffusing it in the air will give the same benefit as drinking the tea by calming the mind and relaxing the body. I am not positive but there are probably candles made with the oils. The plant is used in salves, lotions and I have used it in soaps before. Using it in this form helps with any skin inflammation that I may have such as rashes and leaves my skin smelling fresh with a slight hint of lemon.

As far as safety goes, there are some concerns where lemon balm should not be taken. For example, if you have issues with your thyroid, then do **not** take lemon balm until talking to your doctor. It interacts with the medication and has the possibility of lessening the effects of the medication, which can be a serious problem when it comes to the thyroid. The same goes for medications for glaucoma and sleep disorders. It has a high probability that it will interfere with any prescribed medications for these issues also. Lemon balm should not be given to children under the age of 12 without first talking to a pediatrician.

There are also some side effects that need to be considered before using but these reactions seem to be somewhat rare. Some of those side effects include an upset stomach, headaches, and dizziness. If you experience any of these after using lemon balm, please stop using and talk to a doctor about possible side effects or allergies. It is not recommended to take lemon balm on a long term basis. The recommended time should be three weeks on and one week off if taking on a daily basis.

9

Chamomile

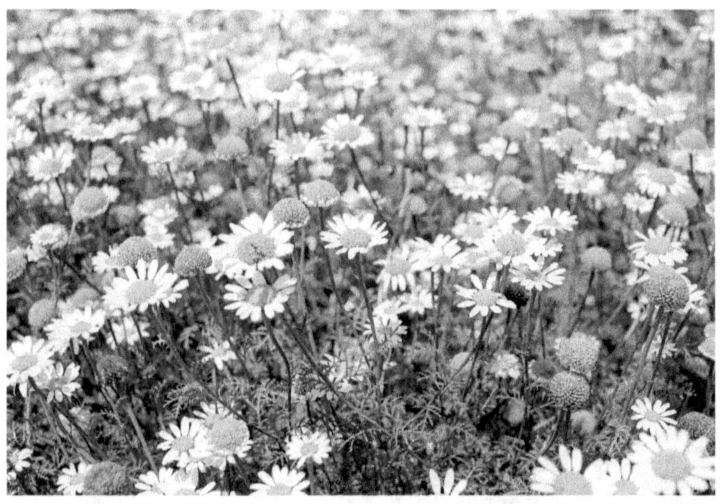

hamomile flowers

Chamomile is a small dainty daisy-like flower that has wispy fern looking leaves. The plant has a faint apple smell and usually grows upright. It has anti-inflammatory and antioxidant properties that have been used for centuries. Ancient texts from Egyptian, Roman and Greek cultures, as early as 5th century B.C.E., mention use of the plant. The texts talk about medical conditions that the plant was used for such as skin conditions, inflammation, wound care, spasms, and as a tea for calming the body. This makes it one of the oldest medicinal plants that has the documentation to back it up yet is still a popular plant that is used in today's society.

There are two types of chamomile available, Roman (*Chamaemelum nobile*) and German (*Matricaria chamomilla*). They differ in not only their appearance, but also in their compound makeup. Roman chamomile has slightly more of a tendency to cause allergic reactions than the German variety but both are still used in the same ways. Most of the research studies have been done with the German variety over the Roman one so a lot of the information is in regards to that particular one.

Chamomile can be used in many forms. There are multiple teas, some blended with other herbs that can be consumed. There is also the essential oil that can be diffused and used in aromatherapy. The oil can be used in personal products or inhaled in a steam bath. Chamomile beer is a thing if herbal beers hold some appeal to you.

The majority of chamomile uses involve tea. It is one of the most popular teas in the world. The benefits of drinking the tea include the ability to calm the nerves, reduce anxiety and depression, and treat sleep problems. There are likewise some digestive complaints that the tea helps with among other ailments. The essential oil can further be used to calm anxiety, help with depression and promote sleep when used in aromatherapy. Not only can the oil be diffused throughout a room but inhaling the steam or using it in a room spray seems to have the same results. Chamomile, usually the Roman variety, is additionally found infused in some bath and body products including shampoo, body lotion, massage oils, bath oils, bath salts, and soap. Tinctures can be made with the flowers and used after sitting and infusing for a few weeks. There are also supplements that can be found in health stores. I have no experience with these and am not sure if they will help with stress and anxiety or if they are used for further ailments that chamomile can help with.

Some of the side effects of chamomile, particularly with the oil, are skin issues such as redness, itching and swelling. There are also allergic reactions that affect a small number of people. However, if you are allergic to asters, ragweed or anything in the daisy family of plants, then chamomile should be avoided. There is a high possibility that you are also allergic to chamomile. Asthma sufferers should also avoid it as it may aggravate asthma. There is a chance of miscarriage if used by pregnant women. So it should be avoided here. Children may be more sensitive to the effects of the herb, a pediatrician should be consulted before use. Some drug interactions could cause issues when working with chamomile. These include medications for diabetes, blood thinner, blood pressure and sleep disorder medications. Check with your doctor and make sure that it is fine to use the herb if you take any prescribed medications.

When it comes to dosage, please follow the recommended doses as prescribed by a physician or that are listed on a label for the product type being used. Always be aware of the form and type of chamomile that you are using. This will help in knowing how potent it can be. Do not take it for a long period of time as the effectiveness may wear off after using it on a regular basis.

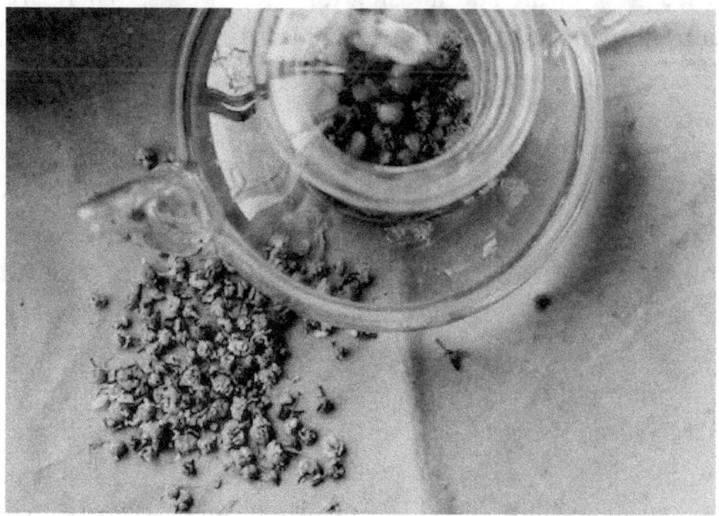

Chamomile tea

10

Conclusion

That's it! These are five plants that have the ability to help manage stress, anxiety, depression, and/or sleep issues. These have less side effects than conventional medications that help with the same problem. Plus most of them also have other conditions that they can help with other than what was mentioned. Being an all natural source, they are not a lab produced chemical which helps keep the prices from being outrageous. The plants listed here have scientific research that back up the claims although there is some research that is still needing verification from more studies. Most of them, if not all, have been used since ancient times. This is only a handful of herbs that can help with symptoms. There are still many more out there that you might have or have not heard of before. I suggest that if you are interested in one (or all) of these plants, that you do your own due diligence and explore the ones that you are interested in before "going all in".

If you are still unsure about using any of these plants, start slow and introduce tea drinking to your routine. You may be surprised by the results and find that it is beneficial. Once that form is found to be helpful, try diffusing some of the oil into the air for a different sensory system. Find which one works best for you and your situation using trial and error. There are enough forms of the herb available between the tea, oils, candles, and bath and body products that there should be something to suit you. If your symptoms are severe though, please consult a physician for assistance with a diagnosis and follow up. Most herbal support is not strong enough to manage severe symptoms. Please also make sure that the precautions are followed for each plant. Most should be run by a licensed physician if you are pregnant, breastfeeding or plan on using it for children. Additionally, all of these have slightly sedative effects, so avoid operating any heavy machinery or participating in any activities that require a heightened sense of being alert. These are basic precautions and safety advice that should be researched and followed up on. Herbs may be all natural but they can still pose a dangerous risk for certain individuals.

If you found this small guide to be helpful, I would appreciate a favorable review being provided on Amazon for the book. Thank you very much!